Homemade Body Butter

A Beginner's Quick Start Guide for Women Over 40, With Sample Recipes and an FAQ copyright © 2022 Stephanie Hinderock

All rights reserved No part of this book may be reproduced, or stored in a retrieval system, or transmitted in any form or by any means, electronic, mechanical, photocopying, recording, or otherwise, without express written permission of the publisher.

Disclaimer

By reading this disclaimer, you are accepting the terms of the disclaimer in full. If you disagree with this disclaimer, please do not read the guide.

All of the content within this guide is provided for informational and educational purposes only, and should not be accepted as independent medical or other professional advice. The author is not a doctor, physician, nurse, mental health provider, or registered nutritionist/dietician. Therefore, using and reading this guide does not establish any form of a physician-patient relationship.

Always consult with a physician or another qualified health provider with any issues or questions you might have regarding any sort of medical condition. Do not ever disregard any qualified professional medical advice or delay seeking that advice because of anything you have read in this guide. The information in this guide is not intended to be any sort of medical advice and should not be used in lieu of any medical advice by a licensed and qualified medical professional.

The information in this guide has been compiled from a variety of known sources. However, the author cannot attest to or guarantee the accuracy of each source and thus should not be held liable for any errors or omissions.

You acknowledge that the publisher of this guide will not be held liable for any loss or damage of any kind incurred as a result of this guide or the reliance on any information provided within this guide. You acknowledge and agree that you assume all risk and responsibility for any action you undertake in response to the information in this guide.

Using this guide does not guarantee any particular result (e.g., weight loss or a cure). By reading this guide, you acknowledge that there are no guarantees to any specific outcome or results you can expect.

All product names, diet plans, or names used in this guide are for identification purposes only and are the property of their respective owners. The use of these names does not imply endorsement. All other trademarks cited herein are the property of their respective owners.

Where applicable, this guide is not intended to be a substitute for the original work of this diet plan and is, at most, a supplement to the original work for this diet plan and never a direct substitute. This guide is a personal expression of the facts of that diet plan.

Where applicable, persons shown in the cover images are stock photography models and the publisher has obtained the rights to use the images through license agreements with third-party stock image companies.

Table of Contents

Introduction	7
What Is Body Butter?	9
How Does It Work?	10
Benefits of Body Butter	10
Common Types Of Body Butter	15
Use Cases	18
How Women Over 40 Starts To Sag and Losing Collagen	22
Pros and Cons of Body Butter	26
Advantages of Homemade Body Butter	26
Disadvantages of Homemade Body Butter	29
Potential Side Effects of Homemade Body Butter	31
Step Guide to Creating a DIY Homemade Butter	34
Safety Tips for Homemade Body Butter	37
Recipes to Try Out	41
Vanilla Bean Body Butter	42
Citrus Bliss Body Butter	43
Rose Petal Body Butter	44
Lavender Mint Body Butter	45
Honey and Oatmeal Body Butter	46
Soothing Chamomile Body Butter	47
Coffee-Infused Body Butter	48
Rosemary and Eucalyptus Body Butter	49
Conclusion	50
FAQs	53
References and Helpful Links	56

Introduction

Are you a woman over 40 looking to nourish your skin naturally? Say goodbye to expensive skincare products that promise miracles but fail to deliver. It's time to discover the power of homemade body butter.

Experience the transformative power of shea butter, coconut oil, and essential oils as they deeply moisturize, rejuvenate, and combat the signs of aging. Take control of your beauty routine and indulge in the self-care you deserve.

Start your skincare transformation today by following our step-by-step instructions and recipes. Discover the joy of creating your nourishing body butter, free from harmful chemicals and tailored to your preferences. Unleash the power of natural ingredients and enjoy the glowing, healthy skin you deserve.

In this Guide, we will talk about the following;

- What is body butter?
- How does it work?
- Benefits of body butter

- Common types of body butter
- Use cases, pros, and cons
- How women over 40 start to sag and lose collagen
- Potential side effects
- Step guide to getting started with homemade body butter
- Safety tips for homemade body butter
- Sample recipes of homemade body butter

Whether you're a seasoned DIY enthusiast or a beginner, making homemade body butter is a rewarding and enjoyable experience every woman over 40 should try. Keep reading for our guide where we'll share more exciting recipes and tips to further enhance your skincare regimen.

What Is Body Butter?

Body butter is a skincare product that is designed to deeply moisturize and nourish the skin. It is typically made with natural fats, such as shea butter or cocoa butter, which have a higher oil concentration compared to lotions. This higher oil content gives body butter a thicker and more luxurious texture.

Unlike body lotion, which has a higher water content and is lighter in texture, body butter provides intense hydration and creates a protective barrier on the skin's surface. The thicker consistency of body butter helps to seal in moisture, making it ideal for individuals with dry skin.

Additionally, body butter tends to have a longer-lasting effect on the skin compared to lotion. Due to its rich formulation, body butter provides a more prolonged period of moisturization, leaving the skin feeling soft, smooth, and nourished.

Another difference between body butter and lotion is how they absorb into the skin. Body butter takes longer to absorb due to its thicker consistency, while lotion absorbs quickly and leaves a lighter, non-greasy feel on the skin. This makes lotions more suitable for daily use, especially during warmer weather or for individuals who prefer a lighter moisturizer.

Overall, the choice between body butter and lotion depends on individual preference and skin needs. Body butter is often favored for drier skin types or areas that require extra hydration, such as elbows, knees, or feet. On the other hand, lotion is a versatile option for everyday moisturization, providing a lightweight feel and quick absorption.

How Does It Work?

Body butter works by creating an oily barrier on the skin that prevents moisture from escaping. This helps to keep your skin soft, smooth, and moisturized throughout the day. The oils in body butter also help to nourish and protect the skin against environmental damage caused by free radicals.

The fatty acids found in body butter act as humectants, which means they attract water from the environment and bind it to your skin. This helps to keep your skin hydrated, even in dry weather conditions.

Benefits of Body Butter

Body butter offers a multitude of benefits for the skin. Here are some of the key benefits:

Moisturizes and Hydrates

Body butter provides exceptional moisturizing and hydration benefits to the skin. Its thick consistency allows for deeper penetration, resulting in lasting hydration and supple skin. The high content of natural butter like shea and cocoa deeply nourishes the skin, protecting it against dryness and reducing the appearance of fine lines and wrinkles.

With regular use, body butter enhances the skin's natural elasticity, leaving it smooth, firm, and glowing. This luxurious product is perfect for those with dry, sensitive, or mature skin, providing a long-lasting and soothing hydration experience.

Protects and Nourishes

The protective and nourishing benefits of body butter are unparalleled. They contain a high concentration of natural oils and fats that penetrate deep into the skin, providing long-lasting moisture. The protective barrier that they create shields the skin from harmful environmental stressors, preventing damage and promoting healthy skin.

With regular use, body butter can improve the appearance of dry, dull skin, leaving it looking glowing and youthful. Their rich texture and luxurious feel make them a pleasure to use, and their natural ingredients make them a safe and effective choice for all skin types. Incorporating body butter into a daily skincare routine is a simple and effective way to achieve beautiful, healthy skin.

Soothes Dryness and Roughness

Body butter is an excellent solution for individuals experiencing dryness and roughness on specific parts of their body, namely elbows, knees, and heels. The product acts as a deeply penetrating moisturizer that provides intense hydration, alleviating these issues. Unlike traditional moisturizers, body butter contains highly concentrated ingredients that efficiently nourish the skin, resulting in long-lasting hydration.

In addition to improving skin texture and appearance, the moisturizing properties of body butter can help prevent skin cracking and flaking. Overall, using body butter can transform dry and rough patches on the body into silky-smooth skin in no time.

Reduces Wrinkles and Signs of Aging

Body butter is a highly nourishing skin care product that effectively reduces wrinkles and signs of aging. Its powerful moisturizing properties are capable of promoting a healthy, youthful, and supple skin texture. Regular use of body butter boosts collagen production, which helps to maintain the elasticity and firmness of the skin.

Additionally, it protects the skin's natural barrier and prevents dehydration, which can lead to premature aging. Enriched with vitamins and minerals, body butter penetrates deeply into the skin, providing long-lasting hydration and nourishment, thus improving the skin's overall health and radiance.

Helps Heal Sunburns, Eczema, and Rashes

Body butter contains moisturizing and emollient properties that can help to alleviate sunburns, eczema, and rashes. Its powerful natural ingredients like shea butter, cocoa butter, and coconut oil have anti-inflammatory and antioxidant properties that soothe and nourish the skin.

These ingredients penetrate deeply into the skin to hydrate and repair damaged skin cells. Body butter can also create a barrier against external factors that can exacerbate skin problems like pollution and UV rays. Regular use of body butter can promote healthy skin and prevent future skin issues from occurring.

Enhances Skin Elasticity

Body butter is a popular skincare product that is rich in essential fatty acids, which are known to improve the skin's elasticity. This property makes it an ideal solution for those looking to reduce stretch marks and promote skin firmness. By deeply moisturizing and nourishing the skin, body butter helps to maintain its natural elasticity, preventing it from becoming dry and prone to cracking.

With regular use, body butter can also help to improve the overall texture and appearance of the skin, leaving it soft, supple, and glowing. The powerful combination of healthy nutrients and minerals in body butter makes it a versatile and effective choice for anyone looking to rejuvenate their skin and achieve a more youthful appearance.

Softens and Smoothes the Skin

Body butter is an excellent way to soften and smoothen the skin, leaving it feeling silky and supple. When used regularly, this luxurious cream deeply moisturizes the skin, providing it with essential nutrients to maintain its health and beauty. Rich in natural oils and butter, body butter penetrates deep into the skin, improving its elasticity and helping to reduce the appearance of fine lines and wrinkles.

Its non-greasy formula leaves no residue, making it perfect for use on the entire body, even in areas prone to dryness. Whether as a daily moisturizer or a special treat after a long day, body butter is an indulgent and effective way to pamper the skin and keep it looking and feeling its best.

Can Benefit Hair and Lips

Body butter is a versatile product that offers numerous benefits for hair and lips. When utilized as a hair conditioner, it penetrates deep into the hair shaft to provide intense hydration, leaving hair silky-smooth and full of shine. Additionally, body butter contains natural emollients and oils that replenish the moisture barrier of the lips, preventing dryness and cracking.

As a result, it helps to maintain soft, supple lips that are free from discomfort. With regular use, body butter is an excellent choice for individuals seeking to boost the health and appearance of their hair and lips.

These are just a few of the many benefits that body butter offers. Its luxurious texture and natural ingredients make it an excellent choice for those looking to pamper and revitalize their skin.

Common Types Of Body Butter

There are several types of body butter available in the market, ranging from commercial products to DIY recipes. The most popular types include:

Shea Butter

Shea butter has become a popular choice for body butter due to its numerous benefits for the skin. It's smooth and easy to apply, making it a go-to choice for those who want to nourish and protect their skin against various environmental factors. In addition to its vitamin-rich properties, Shea butter is also known for its anti-inflammatory and anti-aging properties, making it a great choice for those who want to preserve their skin's youthful appearance.

Its natural hydrating properties can help soothe dry, itchy skin and reduce the appearance of fine lines and wrinkles.

Cocoa Butter

Cocoa butter is a common type of body butter that is rich in fatty acids, antioxidants, and vitamins. It has numerous benefits for the skin, making it an essential ingredient in most skincare products. This butter is widely known for its ability to deeply moisturize the skin and improve its elasticity. It also has a mild chocolatey scent, making it a favorite among chocolate lovers. Cocoa butter is particularly beneficial for mature skin as it helps to reduce the appearance of wrinkles.

The antioxidants present in this butter protect the skin from damage caused by free radicals. It is also effective in reducing the appearance of scars and stretch marks, making it a popular choice for pregnant women. Overall, cocoa butter is an excellent ingredient to incorporate into your daily skincare routine for smooth, nourished, and glowing skin.

Mango Butter

Mango butter is a type of body butter that is often used for its intense hydrating properties. It is a natural fat that is derived from the mango fruit and has a soft, creamy texture that is easy to apply. Unlike other body butter, mango butter does not leave behind an oily residue, making it a good choice for people who don't like greasy moisturizers.

Additionally, mango butter has been known to soothe irritations and reduce redness, making it a popular choice for people with sensitive skin. It is also rich in antioxidants and has been shown to help improve skin clarity and overall health. Due to its many benefits, mango butter is an excellent choice for anyone looking to improve the health and appearance of their skin.

These are just a few of the common types of body butter available in the market. Depending on your specific needs and preferences, you can choose one or combine different types to get the desired results.

Use Cases

Body butter is commonly used to treat various health problems. While it's important to note that scientific evidence may be limited, people have reported positive effects in managing the following conditions:

Dry Skin

Body butter is an excellent solution for individuals struggling with dry and flaky skin. It contains nourishing and emollient ingredients that deeply moisturize and hydrate the skin, leaving it smooth and supple. Unlike regular lotions which often contain a high water content, body butter has a significantly higher concentration of oils and butter, making it more effective in locking in moisture.

Additionally, body butter creates a protective layer on the skin, preventing moisture loss during the day. Its rich texture also means that a little goes a long way, making it a cost-effective solution for individuals with chronic dryness. With regular use, body butter can help to improve the overall appearance and health of the skin, leaving it soft, healthy-looking, and naturally radiant.

Eczema

Shea butter is a popular natural remedy for alleviating eczema symptoms. Its high concentration of essential vitamins and fatty acids makes it incredibly nourishing and moisturizing for the skin. This helps to reduce inflammation, soothe itching, and prevent dryness. Additionally, shea butter has anti-inflammatory properties that can help to soothe red, irritated skin.

When selecting a body butter for eczema treatment, it is important to choose one that is free of artificial fragrances and other harsh chemicals. It is also recommended to do a patch test before applying it all over the affected area to ensure that there is no adverse reaction. By using shea butter regularly, individuals with eczema can experience relief from their symptoms while also promoting overall skin health.

Dermatitis

Body butter can be an effective remedy for relieving dermatitis symptoms. This skin condition causes redness, itching, and inflammation, making it uncomfortable for those who experience it. Fortunately, using body butter, especially those containing shea butter, can help reduce inflammation and calm irritated skin.

Shea butter has anti-inflammatory properties that help soothe skin irritations and prevent further damage. Additionally, body butter provides a moisturizing effect to help restore the skin's natural barrier function. Regular application of body butter can improve the skin's condition and reduce the likelihood of future outbreaks.

Psoriasis

Body butter has been found to effectively provide relief and moisture to psoriasis-affected skin. While it may not be a cure, it can significantly reduce dryness and itchiness, improving the overall comfort of the affected individual. The key to its effectiveness in providing relief lies in its rich composition, which includes ingredients such as shea butter, cocoa butter, and essential oils, all of which have been proven to hydrate and nourish the skin.

The emollient nature of body butter creates a barrier on the skin's surface, sealing in moisture and preventing any further dryness or damage. Additionally, the soothing and anti-inflammatory properties of some of the key ingredients can help reduce the appearance of redness and inflammation associated with psoriasis. Applying body butter consistently and regularly can lead to noticeable improvements in the affected area.

Acne

Body butter is beneficial for individuals with body acne, as it provides hydration without clogging the pores. The moisturizing properties can also help soothe and reduce inflammation. However, it is important to note that body butter is not typically recommended for acne-prone areas of the face, as it can exacerbate breakouts.

It is always best to consult with a dermatologist for personalized advice and to ensure that the product being used is suitable for one's skin type. Additionally, it is important to use a product that is non-comedogenic and free of irritants, fragrances, and dyes to avoid further irritation.

Burns

Body butter, such as shea butter, has been found to aid in the healing process of minor burns. When applied topically, it may help alleviate discomfort by providing a protective layer over damaged skin. In addition, body butter contains natural moisturizing properties which can help prevent dryness and further irritation.

Its high vitamin and mineral content also supplies the skin with essential nutrients that aid in the production of new healthy skin cells. Choosing a body butter with natural ingredients, such as coconut oil or aloe vera, can further enhance its healing benefits. It's important to note that body butter should only be used on minor burns and not on severe or open wounds.

Dandruff

Body butter is effective in soothing dry and flaky scalp conditions like dandruff. Its emollient properties help to hydrate and nourish the scalp while reducing itchiness and irritation. However, it is important to note that not all body butter is suitable for use on the scalp, as some may contain ingredients that could further irritate the skin.

It is recommended to look for hair care products specifically formulated for dandruff relief, but for those who prefer a more natural approach, organic body butter without added fragrances or preservatives could be a viable option. Always conduct a patch test before applying the product to the scalp and discontinue use if any adverse reactions occur.

Remember, individual experiences may vary, and it's crucial to consult with a healthcare professional or dermatologist before using body butter for any specific health concern.

How Women Over 40 Starts To Sag and Losing Collagen

As women age, especially around the age of 40, several changes occur in the body, including the skin. Here are some insights into the effects of aging on women over 40:

Skin Changes

As women approach a certain age, typically around their 40s, they may start to notice significant changes in the appearance and texture of their skin. These changes are primarily due to a decrease in the production of collagen and elastin, which are responsible for maintaining the skin's firmness and elasticity.

As a result, sagging skin, fine lines, and wrinkles become more prominent. Furthermore, the skin tends to become drier and loses its youthful glow, requiring extra care and attention to maintain its vitality and radiance.

Hormonal Shifts

Hormonal shifts during perimenopause, the transitional phase before menopause, commonly occur in a woman's 40s. These fluctuations in hormones, particularly estrogen, and progesterone, can result in a range of symptoms. Hot flashes, characterized by sudden waves of heat and sweating, can be a common occurrence. Mood swings and irritability may also arise due to the hormonal imbalance.

Additionally, changes in skin elasticity and texture may be observed, as decreased estrogen levels affect collagen production. Understanding and managing these hormonal shifts is essential for women navigating this transformative phase of life.

Loss of Muscle Mass

As women age, the natural process of aging can lead to a gradual loss of muscle mass, known as sarcopenia. This decline in muscle tone and strength can affect overall physical fitness and contribute to a decrease in metabolism.

Women over 40 may notice a decrease in muscle mass, making it more important than ever to engage in regular exercise that includes resistance training and strength-building exercises. By prioritizing muscle maintenance and growth, women can help combat the effects of sarcopenia and maintain optimal physical health.

Metabolism Changes

As women age, typically in their 40s and beyond, they may experience a gradual decline in their metabolic rate. This means that their bodies burn calories at a slower pace, making weight management more challenging. To support a healthy metabolism, it becomes crucial to maintain a balanced diet that includes nutrient-dense foods and portion control.

Regular exercise, incorporating both cardiovascular activities and strength training, can also help boost metabolism and preserve muscle mass. Making these lifestyle choices can aid in maintaining a healthy weight and overall well-being.

Bone Health

Women over 40 are at a higher risk of developing osteoporosis, a condition characterized by weak and brittle bones. This is due to the decline in estrogen levels during menopause. It's crucial to prioritize bone health through proper nutrition, weight-bearing exercise, and, if necessary, discuss with a healthcare professional about calcium and vitamin D supplementation.

While these changes may seem overwhelming, it's important to remember that every woman's experience with aging is unique. With proper self-care, a healthy lifestyle, and a positive mindset, women can maintain their beauty, confidence, and well-being as they embrace this new chapter in life.

Pros and Cons of Body Butter

The use of body butter has several pros and cons that must be taken into consideration before use. Below, we will outline some of the key advantages and disadvantages to help you make an informed decision.

Advantages of Homemade Body Butter

Homemade body butter offers a range of advantages, allowing you to customize the ingredients, tailor it to your specific needs, and enjoy the satisfaction of creating a nourishing and luxurious skincare product. Below are some of the key pros associated with body butter:

Natural Ingredients

One of the major advantages of homemade body butter is that it typically contains all-natural ingredients. This makes it a safe and healthy choice for skin care. Natural ingredients are known to be gentler on the skin and help to avoid any harsh chemicals or toxins that may be present in store-bought products. Moreover, the use of natural ingredients in body butter enhances its moisturizing properties, which protect and nourish the skin, resulting in soft and supple skin.

Homemade body butter is also easy to customize, as one can add different natural ingredients based on their skin's needs and preferences. Overall, opting for homemade body butter can significantly improve skin health without any concern for toxic or harmful additives.

Versatile

Homemade body butter is a versatile solution to keep different parts of the body hydrated. Beyond moisturizing the skin, this homemade product can also be applied to the hair, lips, and other facial areas to strengthen and nourish them.

This is because body butter is made with natural ingredients such as shea butter, coconut oil, and essential oils, which are highly moisturizing and packed with vitamins and antioxidants. By using homemade body butter, one can rest assured that they are avoiding synthetic ingredients and harsh chemicals that can be harmful to the skin.

Affordable

Unlike conventional body care products, homemade body butter is an affordable solution for keeping the skin hydrated and healthy. The ingredients needed to make it can typically be found in grocery stores and health food markets at a fraction of the cost of store-bought products. Moreover, these ingredients are often organic, so they are free from harsh chemicals that could negatively affect one's skin.

Customization

Customizing your body butter has many advantages, including the ability to personalize the scent and texture to your liking. However, one of the most significant advantages is the ability to tailor the ingredients to meet your individual needs. Homemade body butter allows you to avoid harmful chemicals and irritants often found in store-bought products, as well as adjust the formulation to address specific skin issues, such as dryness or sensitivity.

By using natural, nourishing ingredients, you can create a luxurious body butter that not only feels wonderful on your skin but also provides long-lasting moisture and nourishment. With homemade body butter, you're able to pamper your skin with a unique blend that suits your personal preferences and needs, leading to healthier, more radiant skin.

These are just some of the many advantages associated with homemade body butter. With its natural ingredients and versatile uses, this product can be a great addition to your skincare routine.

Disadvantages of Homemade Body Butter

Although there are many benefits, homemade body butter has some potential drawbacks. Below are some of the main cons associated with body butter:

Time-Consuming

Crafting homemade body butter can be time-consuming, necessitating an exhaustive procedure of accurately weighing and mixing ingredients. One of the primary inadequacies of the homemade product is the amount of time it consumes to prepare, which extends far beyond merely buying a pre-made solution off the shelf.

While it may allow for customization and experimentation with natural ingredients, the length of time required to create the butter may deter those who require instant results.

Messy

Preparing homemade body butter can be a messy task, requiring the melting of solid ingredients like shea butter and coconut oil before combining them with liquid ingredients like essential oils. This can result in spills and splatters on counters, clothing, and utensils, necessitating thorough cleaning afterward.

Additionally, improperly stored body butter can lead to spoilage or rancidity, potentially causing skin irritation or even infection. While homemade body butter can be a cost-effective alternative to store-bought varieties, the mess, and potential health risks should be taken into consideration before embarking on this DIY project.

Incorrect Proportions

Incorrectly proportioning the ingredients of homemade body butter can have detrimental effects on its effectiveness. Inadequate amounts of key ingredients such as shea butter, coconut oil, and essential oils can alter the final product, resulting in a lack of proper moisturization and nourishment for the skin.

Moreover, an excess of any ingredient can lead to an imbalanced formula, causing irritation and clogging of pores. It is essential to precisely measure each ingredient to ensure the optimal nourishing properties of the body butter.

Unpleasant Smell

When making DIY body butter, it is important to note that some recipes can result in an unpleasant scent that can linger on the skin for a while. This can be attributed to the use of certain ingredients, such as shea butter or cocoa butter, which have distinct natural smells that may not appeal to everyone.

Additionally, homemade body butter may lack the fragrance or masking agents found in store-bought alternatives. While fragrances can be added, they may be too strong or irritate the skin. Therefore, it is crucial to carefully select recipe ingredients and consider the impact of fragrance before making homemade body butter.

Despite these potential drawbacks, homemade body butter is generally safe and beneficial when used correctly.

Potential Side Effects of Homemade Body Butter

While homemade body butter is typically safe, some potential side effects should be taken into consideration.

Allergy

It is important to note that homemade body butter may cause adverse reactions in some individuals. Common side effects include redness, itching, and swelling. These reactions could be caused by an allergy or sensitivity to one or more of the ingredients used in the recipe. If you experience any of these symptoms after using the body butter, it is crucial to discontinue use immediately and seek medical attention.

Consulting with a doctor can help to identify the cause and prevent future reactions. Therefore, it is always advisable to perform a patch test before applying the body butter to your skin. Finally, it is a good practice to check all the ingredients before using them to avoid potential allergies.

Contamination

Contamination can lead to several potential side effects when making homemade body butter. Due to the lack of proper sterilization, bacteria and other harmful microorganisms can grow and potentially cause infections or other complications. These could include skin irritation, rashes, allergic reactions, and even more serious issues such as cellulitis. It is essential to maintain strict hygiene practices when preparing your body butter, including sanitizing tools and thoroughly washing your hands.

Additionally, it is important to only use high-quality, uncontaminated ingredients in your recipe. Taking these steps can help ensure that your homemade body butter is safe and free from potential harm.

Overuse

Overusing homemade body butter can cause a variety of negative effects on the skin. These include oily and sticky skin, which can lead to discomfort and embarrassment. Overuse of body butter can also clog pores and cause breakouts, which can further exacerbate skin problems.

To avoid these potential side effects, individuals should use body butter sparingly and choose lighter formulas that are more easily absorbed into the skin. Additionally, it is important to take note of the ingredients in homemade body butter and ensure that they are safe and non-irritating before use.

When it comes to crafting homemade body butter, it is essential to keep in mind that there are potential drawbacks and side effects. Therefore, it is important to practice caution and adhere to specific instructions when making your own product.

Doing so will ensure that you reap all of the benefits of this wonderful skincare solution without any of the potential risks. With a few simple steps, you will be able to craft quality, nourishing body butter that is sure to leave you with beautiful and glowing skin!

Step Guide to Creating a DIY Homemade Butter

Now that you know the basics of body butter and its potential effects, it's time to get started making your own! Here is a simple step-by-step guide to creating your DIY body butter:

Step 1: Gather your ingredients

Making your body butter is a simple and rewarding process. To start, gather your ingredients: shea butter, coconut oil, and a carrier oil of your choice like almond oil or jojoba oil. These ingredients work together to nourish and moisturize your skin. Shea butter is rich in vitamins and fatty acids that help promote smoothness and elasticity.

Coconut oil is deeply hydrating and has natural antibacterial properties. The carrier oil acts as a base and helps the butter spread easily on your skin. Additionally, you can enhance the fragrance and benefits by adding a few drops of essential oils. With these key ingredients, you can create a luxurious body butter that will leave your skin feeling soft and supple.

Step 2: Melt the ingredients

To melt the shea butter and coconut oil for your body butter, you can follow a simple method. In a double boiler or a heat-safe bowl placed over a pot of simmering water, combine the shea butter and coconut oil. Stir occasionally until both ingredients have completely melted and combined.

This process helps ensure that the ingredients are evenly heated and blended together. The double boiler method is often preferred as it prevents direct heat contact and helps maintain the integrity of the ingredients. You can refer to the sources mentioned above for more detailed instructions and variations in melting the shea butter and coconut oil for your homemade body butter.

Step 3: Add carrier oil and essential oils

Adding carrier oil and essential oils is the next step in making your own body butter. After melting the shea butter and coconut oil, allow the mixture to cool slightly. Then, incorporate your preferred carrier oil and essential oils. Carrier oils enhance the moisturizing effects of the body butter, while essential oils provide fragrance and potential therapeutic benefits. It's important to research the appropriate dilution rates for each essential oil you intend to use.

Step 4: Whip the mixture

After adding the carrier oil and essential oils to the melted shea butter and coconut oil mixture, it's time to whip it up! Using a hand mixer or a stand mixer, set it to medium-high speed and begin whipping the mixture. As you whip, you'll notice the texture transforming from a liquid to a light and fluffy consistency.

This step is crucial as it incorporates air into the body butter, giving it a luxurious and creamy feel. Be patient and continue whipping for several minutes until you achieve the desired consistency. The longer you whip, the lighter and fluffier your body butter will become. Enjoy the process and savor the anticipation of the final result – a nourishing and delightful homemade body butter.

Step 5: Store and enjoy

After creating your homemade body butter, it's time to store and enjoy it! Transfer the body butter into clean, airtight containers like mason jars or glass jars with screw-top lids. It's important to let the body butter cool completely before sealing the containers to avoid condensation and spoilage.

Once sealed, store the containers in a cool, dry place away from direct sunlight. This will help maintain the consistency and extend the shelf life of your body butter. Whenever you're ready to indulge in some self-care, simply open the jar and apply the luxurious body butter onto your skin. Enjoy the moisturizing and nourishing benefits that your homemade creation provides!

Remember, this is a basic recipe, and you can customize it based on your preferences. You can experiment with different carrier oils, and essential oils, and even add natural colors like beetroot powder or cocoa powder for a touch of vibrancy.

Safety Tips for Homemade Body Butter

When making homemade body butter, it's important to take certain safety precautions to ensure the best results. Here are some general safety tips:

Cleanliness

To ensure the safety and quality of homemade body butter, it is crucial to maintain cleanliness throughout the preparation process. This includes thoroughly washing and sanitizing all tools and surfaces involved. Any contamination can be harmful to the user's skin and overall health.

By taking the necessary precautions, individuals can create a safe and effective product for their skin care needs. It is also recommended to store the body butter in a clean, airtight container to prevent any outside bacteria from entering.

Quality Ingredients

Using substandard ingredients while preparing homemade body butter can cause skin irritation and damage rather than providing a moisturizing effect. To ensure the quality of the product, it is crucial to use high-grade oils and butter, mainly organic varieties. Opting for organic ingredients lowers the risk of skin irritation, rashes, and allergies and guarantees the best outcome for the skin.

The use of these ingredients also minimizes the risk of exposure to harmful chemicals or pesticides, keeping skin health and safety a top priority. Therefore, choosing high-quality organic ingredients should be the first and foremost safety tip for anyone intending to prepare homemade body butter.

Patch Test

To ensure safety when using homemade body butter, a patch test on a small area of skin is essential, especially for those with sensitive skin or allergies. This step helps to detect any potential adverse reactions while allowing a person to enjoy the benefits of natural ingredients without harm.

The patch test involves applying a small amount of the body butter to an inconspicuous area and observing any reactions over a few hours or days before using it all over the body. By taking this precautionary measure, one can confidently use homemade body butter without fear of causing unintended harm to the skin.

Allergies and Sensitivities

When making homemade body butter, it is important to take note of any known allergies or sensitivities to specific ingredients. Avoid using any ingredients that may trigger an allergic reaction or irritation. This can include components such as fragrances or chemical preservatives.

Always do a patch test on a small area of the skin before use to ensure there is no adverse reaction. It is also recommended to use organic or natural ingredients as they are usually gentler on the skin. By being mindful of these safety tips, you can enjoy the benefits of homemade body butter without any negative effects.

Sterilized Containers

To ensure the safety of homemade body butter, it is essential to store it in sterilized containers. This prevents bacteria and mold growth. Sterilization can be achieved by washing the containers in hot, soapy water and drying them thoroughly.

It is crucial to sterilize the jars before each use, as even small amounts of bacteria can cause harm to the skin. Taking these simple steps will ensure that your homemade body butter always remains safe to use.

Shelf Life

To ensure the safety of your homemade body butter, it is crucial to be aware of its shelf life. Unlike commercial products, natural ingredients may have a shorter shelf life, which can result in bacterial growth and skin irritation. Adding natural preservatives or storing the body butter in the refrigerator can extend its shelf life and prevent any adverse effects on your skin.

Storage

To ensure that the homemade body butter retains its quality, it is essential to store it in a cool, dry place that is free from direct sunlight. Exposure to extreme temperatures can lead to a change in the consistency, texture, and overall quality of the product. It is critical to avoid drastic temperature fluctuations as they can lead to the butter losing its beneficial properties.

Hence, it is advisable to store the butter in an airtight container in a cupboard or pantry away from any direct heat sources or windows. By taking these safety precautions, the homemade body butter will stay fresh and retain its nourishing properties for longer durations.

Remember, these are general safety precautions for homemade body butter. It's always a good idea to consult specific recipes and sources for additional safety guidelines based on the ingredients used.

Recipes to Try Out

Vanilla Bean Body Butter

Ingredients:

- 1 cup shea butter
- 1/2 cup coconut oil
- 1/2 cup almond oil
- 1 vanilla bean pod (seeds scraped out)
- Optional: a few drops of vanilla essential oil or extract

Instructions:

1. In a double boiler, melt the shea butter, coconut oil, and almond oil together until fully combined.
2. Remove from heat and let it cool slightly.
3. Add the scraped vanilla bean seeds and stir well.
4. If desired, add a few drops of vanilla essential oil or extract for a stronger scent.
5. Transfer the mixture to a clean container and let it cool completely before using.
6. Use it as a luxurious moisturizer on your body.

Citrus Bliss Body Butter

Ingredients:

- 1 cup mango butter
- 1/2 cup jojoba oil
- Zest of 1 orange
- Zest of 1 lemon
- Zest of 1 lime
- 10 drops of sweet orange essential oil
- 5 drops of lemon essential oil
- 5 drops of lime essential oil

Instructions:

1. In a mixing bowl, whip the mango butter until it becomes soft and fluffy.
2. Slowly add the jojoba oil, continuing to whip until well incorporated.
3. Add the zest of orange, lemon, and lime, and mix well.
4. Finally, add the sweet orange, lemon, and lime essential oils, and whip until fully combined.
5. Transfer the body butter to a jar or container and store it in a cool place.
6. Apply to your skin for a refreshing citrus-scented moisturizer.

Rose Petal Body Butter

Ingredients:

- 1 cup cocoa butter
- 1/2 cup rose-infused almond oil
- 10 drops of rose essential oil

Instructions:

1. Melt the cocoa butter in a double boiler until fully liquid.
2. Remove from heat and let it cool for a few minutes.
3. Add the rose-infused almond oil and rose essential oil, and stir well.
4. Allow the mixture to cool completely before placing it in the refrigerator for about an hour.
5. Once the mixture has solidified but is still soft, use a hand mixer or stand mixer to whip it into a fluffy texture.
6. Transfer the whipped body butter to a jar or container and use as desired.

Lavender Mint Body Butter

Ingredients:

- 1 cup shea butter
- 1/2 cup coconut oil
- 1/2 cup almond oil
- 10 drops of lavender essential oil
- 5 drops of peppermint essential oil

Instructions:

1. In a double boiler, melt the shea butter, coconut oil, and almond oil together until fully combined.
2. Remove from heat and let it cool for a few minutes.
3. Add the lavender and peppermint essential oils and stir well.
4. Allow the mixture to cool completely before using a hand mixer or stand mixer to whip it into a creamy consistency.
5. Transfer the whipped body butter to a jar or container and store it in a cool place.
6. Apply to your skin for a soothing and refreshing moisturizer.

Honey and Oatmeal Body Butter

Ingredients:

- 1 cup shea butter
- 1/2 cup cocoa butter
- 1/2 cup coconut oil
- 1/4 cup honey
- 1/4 cup ground oatmeal

Instructions:

1. In a double boiler, melt the shea butter, cocoa butter, and coconut oil until fully melted and well combined.
2. Remove from heat and let it cool for a few minutes.
3. Stir in the honey and ground oatmeal until evenly distributed.
4. Allow the mixture to cool completely before using a hand mixer or stand mixer to whip it into a fluffy texture.
5. Transfer the whipped body butter to a jar or container and store it in a cool place.
6. Apply to your skin for a nourishing and exfoliating moisturizer.

Soothing Chamomile Body Butter

Ingredients:

- 1 cup shea butter
- 1/2 cup almond oil
- 10 drops of chamomile essential oil

Instructions:

1. Melt the shea butter in a double boiler until fully liquid.
2. Remove from heat and let it cool for a few minutes.
3. Add the almond oil and chamomile essential oil, stirring well.
4. Allow the mixture to cool completely before placing it in the refrigerator for about an hour.
5. After it has solidified but is still soft, whip it into a fluffy texture using a hand mixer or stand mixer.
6. Transfer the whipped body butter to a jar or container and use as desired.

Coffee-Infused Body Butter

Ingredients:

- 1 cup cocoa butter
- 1/2 cup coconut oil
- 1/4 cup ground coffee

Instructions:

1. Melt the cocoa butter and coconut oil in a double boiler.
2. Add the ground coffee and stir well.
3. Strain the mixture to remove the coffee grounds.
4. Let the mixture cool and solidify, then whip it into a fluffy texture.
5. Transfer to a container and use as an invigorating morning moisturizer.

Rosemary and Eucalyptus Body Butter

Ingredients:

- 1 cup shea butter
- 1/2 cup almond oil
- 10 drops rosemary essential oil
- 5 drops of eucalyptus essential oil

Instructions:

1. Melt the shea butter using a double boiler.
2. Remove from heat and add the almond oil, then the rosemary and eucalyptus essential oils, stirring until well combined.
3. Let it cool and harden, then whip the mixture until it's light and fluffy.
4. Transfer to a container and use as a refreshing moisturizer.

Remember, you can adjust these recipes to your preferences, and try combining different essential oils for a personalized scent! Enjoy the process of making your nourishing body butter.

Conclusion

Congratulations, fabulous women over 40! You've made it to the end of our homemade body butter guide, and we hope you're feeling inspired and ready to embark on your journey to luxurious, youthful skin. Throughout this guide, we have explored various recipes and tips to help you create your very own nourishing body butter. Now, let's wrap it all up with some final insights and encouragement to keep you motivated on this wonderful self-care adventure.

Creating your homemade body butter is not just about pampering yourself; it's a powerful act of self-love and empowerment. As we age, our skin requires extra attention and care, and what better way to provide that than by using natural, high-quality ingredients that you carefully choose yourself? By taking control of what goes onto your skin, you're embracing your inner goddess and embracing the beauty that comes with age.

One of the key benefits of homemade body butter is that it allows you to tailor the recipe to your specific needs. Whether you're looking to combat dryness, reduce the appearance of fine lines, or simply indulge in a little self-indulgence, there's a body butter recipe out there for you. Experiment with different combinations of oils, butter, and essential oils to find the perfect blend that suits your unique skin type and preferences.

The recipes we've explored offer a variety of options, from a whipped shea butter base to coconut oil-infused concoctions. Each ingredient brings its own set of benefits to the table. Shea butter is deeply moisturizing and rich in vitamins, while coconut oil provides antibacterial properties and a delicious tropical scent. Don't forget the power of essential oils, which not only add fragrance but also bring their skin-loving properties to the mix.

But homemade body butter isn't just about the final product; it's about the process itself. Taking the time to gather your ingredients, melt them together, and whip them into a creamy texture is a therapeutic experience in itself. Embrace this ritual as a mindful practice, allowing yourself to fully indulge in the moment and savor the anticipation of the luxurious treat you're about to create.

Now, let's talk about the remarkable results you can expect from using your homemade body butter. With regular use, you'll notice that your skin becomes softer, smoother, and more supple. Fine lines may appear diminished, and any dry patches will be a thing of the past. The nourishing ingredients penetrate deep into the skin, promoting cellular regeneration and giving your body the love and care it deserves.

But beyond the physical benefits, using homemade body butter is a beautiful act of self-care that transcends age. It's a reminder that no matter how busy life gets or how many candles are on our birthday cake, we are worthy of love, attention, and pampering. So take that extra five minutes each day to massage your homemade body butter into your skin, and let it be a loving reminder of your worth and beauty.

Remember, dear women over 40, age is just a number. Your wisdom, grace, and confidence make you shine from within. Embrace your journey and wear your skin proudly. Let your homemade body butter be a testament to your self-love and a daily reminder to prioritize your well-being.

So, grab your saucepan, gather your ingredients, and dive into the world of homemade body butter. Get creative, experiment, and have fun along the way. Treat yourself to a little self-indulgence and enjoy the process of caring for your skin like never before.

Here's to radiant skin, boundless confidence, and the joy of self-care at every age. You deserve it!

FAQs

What is body butter?

Body butter is a nourishing and moisturizing skincare product that is typically made from a combination of natural plant oils, butter, and herbs. It has a thick and creamy texture that melts upon contact with the skin, providing deep hydration and leaving a smooth and soft feeling.

How is body butter different from lotions?

The main difference between body butter and lotions lies in their composition. Body butter is usually made with a higher concentration of oils and butter, resulting in a thicker consistency and more intense moisturization. Lotions, on the other hand, contain more water and are lighter in texture.

What are the benefits of using homemade body butter?

Homemade body butter offers several benefits for your skin. It helps to lock in moisture, soothe dry and irritated skin, improve skin elasticity, and promote a healthy and youthful appearance. It also allows you to customize the ingredients according to your skin's specific needs and preferences.

Can I use body butter on all skin types?

Yes, body butter can be used on all skin types, including dry, normal, sensitive, and mature skin. However, it's important to choose ingredients that suit your skin's needs. For example, those with oily or acne-prone skin may prefer lighter oils like grapeseed or jojoba, while drier skin types may benefit from heavier butter like shea or cocoa butter.

How do I make my own homemade body butter?

Making homemade body butter is a fun and rewarding process. Start by melting a combination of oils and butter, such as shea butter, cocoa butter, and coconut oil, over low heat. Once melted, allow the mixture to cool slightly before adding any desired essential oils or fragrances. Finally, whip the mixture until it reaches a light and fluffy consistency. You can find detailed recipes and guides online to help you get started.

How long does homemade body butter last?

The shelf life of homemade body butter can vary depending on the ingredients used and the storage conditions. Generally, body butter made with natural preservatives like vitamin E oil or rosemary extract can last for several months to a year. It's important to store your body butter in a cool and dry place to prevent spoilage and maintain its quality.

Can I use homemade body butter on my face?

While body butter is primarily formulated for use on the body, it can also be used on the face with caution. Despite this fact, do know that facial skin is more delicate and prone to breakouts, so it's essential to choose ingredients that are non-comedogenic and suitable for facial use. Before applying homemade body butter to your face, it is best to get the opinion of a dermatologist, especially if you have acne-prone skin or skin that is easily irritated.

References and Helpful Links

Millar, H. (2022, February 7). What to know about body butter and body lotion. https://www.medicalnewstoday.com/articles/body-butter-vs-lotion

11 benefits of using natural body butter. (2017, September 1). Magical Tree Skincare. https://www.magical-tree.com/blogs/our-story/11-benefits-of-using-natural-body-butters

Ghati, M. (2023, March 28). Can Body Butter Be Used On Face | Clean Beauty Coach. CLEAN BEAUTY COACH. https://cleanbeautycoach.com/can-body-butter-be-used-on-face/

Bharat, D. (2021b, August 10). Body Butter: Splendid Benefits To Soothe Dry Skin And The Different Types. Netmeds. https://www.netmeds.com/health-library/post/body-butter-splendid-benefits-to-soothe-dry-skin-and-the-different-types

Clarke, A. (2019, January 30). Should you use shea butter for eczema? Healthline. https://www.healthline.com/health/shea-butter-for-eczema

Schneider, K. (2022, December 14). 6 Incredible benefits of shea Butter. Cleveland Clinic. https://health.clevelandclinic.org/shea-butter-benefits/

Bharat, D. (2021, August 10). Body Butter: Splendid Benefits To Soothe Dry Skin And The Different Types. Netmeds.

https://www.netmeds.com/health-library/post/body-butter-splendid-benefits-to-soothe-dry-skin-and-the-different-types

www.ingramcontent.com/pod-product-compliance
Lightning Source LLC
LaVergne TN
LVHW012038060526
838201LV00061B/4664